Understanding Body Weight

- Weight Management Series

Volume 2

Excerpt from Adopting a healthy lifestyle (1-884711-34-0)

Understanding Body Weight

Weight Management Series

C.T. Pam

Copyright © 2013 by C. T. Pam

Published and printed in the United States by Innovative Publishers, Inc., Boston, Massachusetts.

Library of Congress Control Number: 2012922835

1-884711-70-7 978-1-884711-70-1 Paperback

Also available in the following formats
1-884711-71-5 978-1-884711-71-8 Kindle
1-884711-72-3 978-1-884711-72-5 Hardback
1-884711-73-1 978-1-884711-73-2 AudioBook
1-884711-74-X 978-1-884711-74-9 iBook
1-884711-75-8 978-1-884711-75-6 Nook

Designations used by companies to distinguish their products are often claimed as trademarks. In all instances where Innovative Publishers Inc. is aware of the claim, the product name appears in initial capital or all capital letters. Readers, however, should contact the appropriate companies for more complete information regarding trademarks and registration.

No part of this publication may be reproduced, stored in a retrieval system, or transmitted in any form or by any means, electronic, mechanical, photocopying, recording, scanning, or otherwise except as permitted under Section 107 or 108 of the 1976 United States Copyright Act, without either the prior written permission of the publisher, or authorization through payment of the appropriate per copy fee to the Copyright Clearance Center, 222 Rosewood Dr., Danvers, MA 01923, 978 – 750 – 8400, fax 978 – 646 – 8600, or on the web at www.copyright.com. Requests to the publisher for permission should be addressed to the Permissions Department, Innovative Publishers Inc., PO Box 300446, Boston, MA 02130, or online at http://innovative-publishers.com.

The information contained in this book is not intended to serve as a replacement for professional medical advice. Any use of the information in this book is that the reader's discretion. The author and the publisher specifically disclaim any and all liability arising directly or indirectly from the use or application of any information contained in this book. A healthcare professional should be consulted regarding your specific situation. For general information about our other products and services, please contact our customer care department within the United States. Specific contact information can be found online at http://innovative-publishers.com.

Printed in the United States of America

10 9 8 7 6 5 4 3 2 1 13 14 15 16

First edition, February 2013

All rights reserved under International and Pan-American Copyright Conventions.

Limit of Liability/Disclaimer of Warranty: While the publisher and author have used their best efforts in preparing this book, they make no representations or warranties with respect to the accuracy or completeness of the contents of this book and specifically disclaim any implied warranties or merchantability of fitness for a particular purpose. While all attempts have been made to verify information, neither the author or the publisher nor the marketing agents assumes any responsibility for errors, omissions, or contrary interpretation of the subject matter whatever the circumstances. No warranty may be created or extended by sales representatives or written sales materials. The advice and strategies contained herein may not be suitable for your situation. You should consult with a professional where appropriate. Neither the publisher nor the author shall be liable for any loss of profit or any commercial damages, including but not limited to special, incidental, consequential, or other damages.

For general information on our other products and services or for technical support, please contact our technical support within the United States at pub@innovative-publishers.com online at http://innovative-publishers.com.

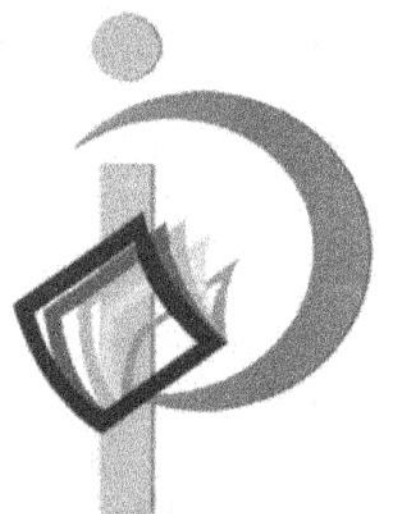

Table of contents

Introduction to Weight Management

With the rapid rate at which obesity has spread over the last couple of decades, the importance of weight management programs has also grown as a consequence. Weight management program refers to all those activities that help an individual to either gain weight, lose weight or even to maintain it at the current level. In any of these goals, a weight management program targets increasing or maintaining the amount of lean muscle mass while decreasing the body fat percentage. Any other way of losing or gaining weight will be unhealthy in one aspect or another and may compromise health in the short term, but definitely in the long run.

Body Composition

Our body comprises of different components, namely fat, lean muscle, water, bones, organs etc. Each of them contributes to the total body weight. For each and every individual each of these constituent elements is present in different proportions. The ratio in which this distribution is present in any individual is called body composition. In the context of weight management, the division is done into two categories – fat mass and fat free mass. A healthy body composition is one in which the fat mass is low and fat free mass is higher. Through different weight management programs it is attempted to alter body composition in a manner that it boosts good health.

There are many techniques and methods to determine body composition. With technological advancements newer and more accurate equipments are available for performing body composition analysis. Traditional techniques such as skin fold measurements are easy to implement but have limited accuracy. Newer technologies such as ultrasound and bioelectric impedance analysis help in doing body composition analysis using simple and portable machines that give extremely accurate results as well. These different methods determine not only the amount of fat and lean muscle tissue but also provide a segmental analysis so that appropriate intervention strategies can be planned as part of the weight management program.

Doing body composition analysis on a regular basis should be included as part of any weight management strategy since it will help in monitoring the alterations taking place in the body as a result of the program. Since the body is undergoing change on a regular basis it is imperative that the program should also change accordingly. A program that was designed for the individual who weighed say 240 pounds will need to be changed when the person loses weight and weighs 200 pounds now. Body composition analysis also provides information on whether the weight loss is happening in a healthy manner or not. In case the weight loss happens at the expense of lean muscle or water then changes need to be done in the program so that these components can be restored to normal levels and fat loss targeted by introducing appropriate changes. A number of new age weight loss methods as well as gadgets are able to provide good results in terms of weight loss but they do it at the expense of good health. Doing a simple body composition analysis will reveal the true nature of these unhealthy methods and systems. Most new technologies also provide information on metabolic rate which is directly correlated the amount of lean mass in the body. Greater the lean mass higher will be the energy that is required by the body to maintain it. The measurement of metabolic rate helps in designing the exercise program as well as the calorie intake required as part of the diet & nutrition plan. Since the needs and requirement of each and every individual are different, the weight management strategy has to be necessarily different as well. Body composition analysis is the first step in designing a weight management program and should thereafter be done on a regular basis.

Problems with adverse body composition

A body composition analysis that reveals high fat percentage in comparison to lean muscle mass percentage points to obesity. Obesity is a modern day lifestyle disease that is essentially a silent killer. It indirectly leads to other physical as well as mental disorders, ailments and diseases that later on deplete the quality of life of the individual and in certain cases may even lead to death. The most common ailments that accompany obesity include type-2 diabetes, hypertension, cardiovascular & coronary artery disease, metabolic syndrome polycystic ovary syndrome and Dyslipidemia. Obesity also leads to gastrointestinal issues such as Cholelithiasis, GERD or Gastroesophageal Reflex Disease, Fatty Liver Disease, Colon Cancer and Hernia; genitourinary problems include erectile dysfunction, renal failure, incontinence and hypogonadism; Respiratory problems include sleep apnea, Hypoventilation syndrome and dyspnea. Apart from these physical ailments obesity also leads to psychological problems that arise from a diminished self confidence and if left unchecked may even lead to chronic depression.

Causes of Obesity

Obesity is caused by an energy intake in the form of diet that is not balanced by equivalent amount of physical activity. The basic law of conservation of energy cannot be violated at any cost and hence, energy excess will lead to weight gain while energy deficit will lead to weight loss. Energy input into the body is through the food that we eat. Energy output is the sum of a number of parameters that include – energy expended through physical exercise, energy spent in activities performed in daily life, basal metabolic rate or the energy required by the body to perform essential body functions such as respiration and digestion; in addition there are a few other parameters such as *thermic effect of food* and *adaptive thermogenesis* that add onto energy output but only in relatively small amounts. It is when the energy input becomes greater than energy output that the body starts storing this excess energy in the form of body fat. Some amount of fat is essential for efficient body functioning but when the fat percentage goes above certain levels it leads to obesity and consequently a host of other disorders and diseases.

This energy imbalance is the objective reason behind obesity but it is important to understand the underlying reasons why this imbalance is created. Imbalanced diet and sedentary lifestyle are the primary causes which get accentuated as a result of numerous personal, social, cultural and familial issues. Genetics and medical conditions also contribute towards increasing the fat mass in an individual. While most parameters seem to be alterable, some of these parameters may not seem to be in control of the individual and a situation of helplessness may be experienced. However, there are ways and means to counter any of these issues that gradually lead to weight loss in a healthy manner.

Genetic factors and Body Type

As mentioned above certain parameters that influence body composition cannot be modified. Genetic predisposition is one such parameter. Genetics define the body type of an individual which then affects the way in which the body reacts to a certain lifestyle and also to any alteration that is forced on this lifestyle. There are different classification techniques for differentiating between different body types.

1. The ancient Indian science of *Ayurveda* uses a classification method based on energy patterns or types. It is believed as per *Ayurveda* that the universe comprises of five basic elements – space, air, water, fire and earth. A combination of these basic elements is responsible for defining the human physiology. The basis of classification therefore is on the basis of energy patterns or *doshas* which comprise of one or more of these elements. The three *doshas – vata, pitta* and *kapha* define the person's physiology and all *Ayurvedic* treatments start from the identification of the *dosha* and identifying the imbalance in the *dosha* pattern. Once this is done remedial solution can be prescribed the aim of which is to restore the balance in the elements.
2. The second classification technique is based on the metabolic type. Under this classification technique the basis of differentiation between body types is the dominating gland in the endocrine system. It is believed that the biochemical reactions happening in the body of the individual are influenced and controlled by the dominating gland. This dominance of one particular gland over the others is built into the genetic structure and has a significant impact on the metabolic processes in the body. These metabolic processes take up raw materials such as carbohydrates, fats, proteins in different proportions and occur in the presence of catalysts that are available through micronutrients such as minerals and vitamins. The difference in proportions of raw material

utilized is due to the functioning differences between these glands of the endocrine system. The classification is done into 4 main categories – adrenal (controls reaction to environmental stresses and dangers), gonad (controls reproduction and growth), thyroid (controls metabolism) and pituitary (control the secretion of all glands) depending upon the dominating gland. Different diets and exercise routines are recommended for different body types.

3. The third classification technique and most commonly used in the context of weight management programs is on the basis of Somatotype. The system is based on identifying the association between psychological behavior patterns or temperament with the body structure of the individual. Under this system it is believed that the characteristic behavioral patterns as exhibited by an individual are typical of his or her own body type to a significantly large extent. The body type as in other classification systems is genetically predetermined. People having a similar body type are expected to show similar behavioral traits under this system. The system of classification is on the basis of the 3 elements or Somatotypes that are named after cell groups known as *germinal epithelium* formed during the growth of the embryo in the womb. The three Somatotypes are named after the three germ layers - *mesoderm, endoderm* and *ectoderm* and are therefore called Mesomorph, Endomorph and Ectomorph respectively. Mesomorphs are characterized by a predominance of lean muscle, connective tissues and bone; Endomorphs are characterized by a predominant roundness & softness in the different parts of the body as a consequence of excess body fat; Ectomorphs are characterized by fragility & linearity and are therefore possess frail and weak body structures which are devoid of fat as well as lean muscle. An individual may not necessarily be a pure Somatotype and can be a combination of one or more of these Somatotypes.

These body types are not inflexible to change arising from application of stimulus in the form of exercise and diet. Not each and every one possesses a dream body shape and structure by birth. Similarly, not everyone who has the nature predisposition to a good physique is able to maintain it. The genetic code embedded into our body in the form of body type plays a significant role in determining our body shape but it is not the only parameter. It is true that an Ectomorph may ingest large number of calories as part of diet and may perform rigorous strength training routines but still may find it difficult to add an extra pound of weight. Similarly, an endomorph may perform long duration cardiovascular workouts but still may not be able to shed those extra pounds of fat stored in the body. However, genetic predisposition only indicates the difficulty to create changes; nowhere does it mention that it is impossible. Moreover, in most cases an individual is a combination of Somatotypes which makes it possible to create changes in one direction or the other depending upon the requirement. It is therefore of utmost importance to identify the body type and the goals before designing an exercise program and diet plan. Once this identification has been done, adherence to a scientifically designed weight management program will lead to achievement of the desired targets that have been set.

Components of weight management program

A healthy weight management program should be based on the four pillars of wellness – physical fitness, balanced diet & nutrition, rest & relaxation and mental attitude. A balance between all the four components is crucial for the success of a weight management program. A good fitness routine which is not accompanied by an appropriate diet will not help the individual trying to lose weight. Similarly, a person who does not have the right mental frame of mind will find it extremely difficult to adhere to certain basic restrictions that such a program may impose; as a result of which the whole program fails. A weight management program needs to be customized according the needs and goals of the individual. This customization needs to be reflected in all the components as well. In case even one of them is not in sync it can derail the whole program itself.

Balanced diet & nutrition

A good balanced and nutritious diet is paramount to the success of a weight management program. Not only should it provide the right amount of energy depending upon the goals of the program, it should also provide the necessary micronutrients in adequate quantities for long term sustainable weight loss and overall health. A balanced diet incorporates energy compounds such as carbohydrates, fats and proteins, micronutrients such as vitamins and minerals as well as fiber and water in adequate quantities. As mentioned before the quantity and proportion of the main energy compounds depends on the goal of the program while micronutrients should be available to the body as per standard guidelines such as DV (Daily Value), RDA (Recommended Dietary Allowance) and EAR (Estimated Average Requirement).

In case the goal is to lose weight then an energy deficit needs to be created in a way that energy intake is less than energy output. This may involve reducing the quantities of the energy compounds from the normal diet and vice versa in case weight gain is the goal. As part of a weight management diet plan identifying the calorie content of meals is extremely crucial. To lose one pound of fat, a deficit of 3,500 calories needs to be created. This can be done by ensuring a regular deficit of 500 calories per day throughout the week. A gradual weight loss rate of one to two pounds per week is ideal for the body since it gets time to adapt to the changed conditions. Moreover, gradual weight loss ensures that there is least amount of muscle loss that happens as part of the weight loss process. This is where the efficacy of crash diets or very low calorie diets is questioned. Apart from loss of muscle tissue they cause micronutrient deficiency extremely dangerous to overall health. Certain research studies also confirm that such diets in fact may lead to fat gain since the body experiences starvation and tends to preserve the energy dense compounds for later utilization. This is done at the expense of lean muscle tissue which is difficult to maintain in the body.

In general any meal should include around 55 to 60% energy being provided through carbohydrates, 25 to 30% energy through fats and approximately 10 to 20% through proteins. This principally ensures that while all the energy requirements are met, nourishment of the body is not compromised upon. Even in case an energy deficit is required for losing weight it created in such a way that all nutrients including fats are available to the body for essential functions that need to be performed for healthy a mind & body.

Once the energy requirements have been calculated the next step in the preparation of a balanced diet plan is identification of the meals and meal content. By identification of the meals, it is intended to finalize the meal frequency and the meal timings such that they can be incorporated in the lifestyle in an easy manner. Too many alteration in the existing pattern of life make the adherence to the plan that much more difficult. Therefore, a diet plan should be designed taking into consideration the individual's lifestyle and preferences. In this context the question of meal frequency becomes a pertinent one. The three meal plan has been ingrained into modern day diets since it is conveniently adopted into work life pattern. It may not necessarily be as good and efficient for overall health as well as for weight loss in comparison to a high frequency diet plan such as a 6 meal plan.

Our body requires energy at a particular rate; this rate is defined by our metabolic rate but there may be spikes in demand such as the post exercise period. Clearly, the body does not require energy at the rate at which we eat and the rate at which the energy is released in our body upon digestion of food. In such a situation the excess energy needs to be stored in the body to be utilized at a later stage. The body can do it in the form of glycogen in the liver and muscles but once these limited space stores are filled up then it converts the extra energy into fat which can be stored all over the body. Secondly, whenever a heavy meal is consumed the insulin spike that occurs upon increase in glucose level in the blood, stays on for a longer period of time. In a similar manner this also results in storage of carbohydrates initially as glycogen but later on as fat. Smaller meals ensure that the body gets energy at a rate commensurate to its requirements so that it does not have to convert and store it as body fat. A high frequency 6 meal plan aids in this process of immediate utilization.

The other factor is the proportion of energy that is derived from stored energy reserves versus that derived from food that has been consume in the recent past. The body stores energy compounds like glucose in the blood, glycogen or long chain glucose molecules in the liver and muscles. And fat in the adipose tissue. Whenever the requirement for energy arises the body meets it through one of these sources. When extra carbohydrates are ingested as part of the meal the body stops utilizing the fat stored in the body, on top of this, the extra carbohydrate gets converted into fat. In a high frequency meal plan, the amount of carbohydrates consumed in any meal is limited, which prevents prolonged insulin spike from occurring. This helps in preventing conversion of carbohydrates into fat and also helps in utilizing stored fat for meeting energy requirement.

As part of weight management programs high frequency smaller meals are often suggested due to the aforementioned reasons. The other psychological advantages offered by these plans are beneficial in ensuring adherence during the initial difficult periods of change. By trimming down meal quantities and increasing frequency, cravings that lead to unplanned eating can be prevented. Since, as part of the meal itself there are many meals, the meal content is pre-planned and hence, the chances of eating something unhealthy out of the diet plan are reduce. Uncontrolled hunger pangs are also not experienced since the gap between meals is shorter. This has a dual advantage – apart from preventing binge eating it also helps in avoiding overeating during the main meals. The effect of frequent meals on metabolism has also been seen to be positive in nature. By eating frequent meals, the body is not allowed to go onto starvation mode and thereby the metabolism is maintained at a high since there it is made to experience a near constant availability of food and energy. Increased metabolism helps in burning the extra fat reserves in the body and hence helps in losing weight in a desirable manner. In summary, a high frequency smaller meal plan seems to be much more effective in reducing body fat percentage in comparison to the modern day three meal plan. This loss in fat percentage is ideal for weight loss as well as weight gain. Hence such a meal plan can be made an integral part of any weight management program.

Physical exercise as part of weight management plan

The second pillar in a healthy weight management program is regular physical exercise at the right intensity. It helps in increasing the energy output to create the deficit that is essential for weight loss to take place. In case weight gain is the goal, exercise provides stimulus forcing the body to grow to meet the additional demands placed on it. Whatever the goals may be, like a healthy weight management plan, a healthy exercise routine should include all the components – cardiovascular endurance, muscular endurance, muscular strength and flexibility.

1. Cardiovascular endurance exercises include all those exercises that involve repetitive movement of large muscle groups at a heart rate greater than resting heart rate. Exercises include running, jogging, swimming, cycling, rowing etc. The role of the cardiovascular system is to ensure efficient delivery of oxygen to different parts of the body. Performing regular cardio exercises not only improves the delivery mechanism of oxygen but also helps improve the efficiency of the vascular system and the exercising muscles to take up and utilize the oxygen delivered. Chronic adaptations as a result of cardio activities help in preventing cardiovascular and coronary artery diseases, metabolic disorders such as diabetes and metabolic syndrome and may also help in preventing certain forms of cancer.
2. Muscular endurance exercises help improve the endurance of different muscle groups in the body. Numerous activities of daily life involve repeated movements to be performed of a particular type and therefore utilize a particular muscle group. Improved muscular endurance helps in performing these movements without experiencing too much fatigue in the exercising muscle.
3. Muscular strength is the ability of a particular muscle to lift heavy loads. In daily life, the requirement to lift and carry heavy load often arises but infrequently. If the body is deconditioned to perform such a movement then there is risk of injury. Strength training exercises help in increasing lean muscle tissue in the body as well as improves the quality of

bone health by strengthening them. In such a manner it helps in performing activities of daily life.

4. Flexibility refers to pain free range of motion around a joint. This is one of the most neglected aspects of fitness and as age progresses it becomes the most important component. Flexibility training in the form of static stretches held for moderate to long durations helps in improving flexibility which then reduced the risk of injuries.

All these components of exercise are important in the context of weight management but more emphasis is directed towards exercises such as cardiovascular workouts. These exercises increase the heart rate in such a manner that the extra demands placed on the body force it to rely on stored energy reserves in the body. By careful planning of diet and intensity of workout it is possible to selectively utilize fat stored in the body for meeting the energy requirements. A balanced routine should include 40 minutes of moderate intensity aerobic activity for 3 to 4 times a week, strength training or resistance training of all the muscle groups at least twice a week and static stretching to improve flexibility should also be incorporated at least 2 to 3 times a week. Such a balanced workout leads to weight loss as well as improves overall physical fitness.

Rest & Relaxation

It is important to understand that the actual growth and development of the body does not take place while exercise is being performed. Exercise only provides the stimulus required for growth and development of tissues. The other ingredients that ensure that the purpose is fulfilled are balanced & nutritious diet and rest & relaxation. Post exercise when the body rests and is provided energy and nutrition is the time when the actual growth happens. At this stage the energy requirements should be met from within the fat stores for weight loss to take place. In case this is not done, the body will strip lean muscle tissue to meet the demands post by exercise. Also, in case enough rest is not provided to the body, the chance of overtraining leading to injury increases manifold. Adequate amount of rest and relaxation also helps in maintaining hormonal balance in the body. This is also crucial for healthy weight management.

Mental attitude

A perfectly designed diet plan or a perfectly designed exercise routine is of no use if the individual for whom it is designed is not able to adhere to it. This is where the role of a positive mental attitude comes into picture. Psychological factors play an important role in weight management than is generally imagined. In fact adherence to any plan is solely dependent on the attitude a person carries towards the lifestyle alteration that is being imposed as part of the plan. In case the weight management program is looked at as a set of limitations or restrictions that is forced, the chances of adherence in the short run as well as over a period of time diminish significantly. On the contrary an individual adopting a positive attitude looks at the program as a new positive lifestyle which is embraced with vigour and excitement.

Yoga for weight management

'Yoga' is derived from '*yuj*' in Sanskrit which means 'to unite'. Originating in ancient India, it is a unique combination of mental, physical as well as spiritual disciplines. This union that yoga refers to is the union of the individual with the universal. Yoga is believed to have originated more than 25,000 years ago and contrary to common knowledge it is not just a sequence of poses and postures for improving health and fitness. It is an ancient science that includes tools such as *pranayama* or breathing methods and techniques, meditation also called *dhyana* and finally physical postures or *asanas*.

The modern form of yoga is believed to have begun with Parliament of Religions convened in Chicago in the year 1893. In the convention *Swami Vivekanand* had a deep impact on the thinking of the audience. In subsequent tours in the United States he promoted various aspects of yoga. These talks and lectures led to yoga shedding the tag of a purely religious practice and being accepted by the western world. In the years since then health benefits emanating through regular yogic practices have been researched, documented and published all over the world. It is estimated that in the US alone more than 25 million people practice yoga on a regular basis.

The myriad benefits of yoga include physiological benefits such as improved flexibility, increased strength, better posture, weight loss, effective breathing, stronger immune system, improved bone strength and improvement in medical conditions such as migraine and insomnia; psychological benefits include stress relief, greater awareness, improved energy levels and an overall feeling of inner peace. Yoga is quite efficient in weight loss as well. It advocates a multi dimensional approach that incorporates physical, emotional and spiritual components and does not superficially work on eliminating the symptoms alone. The root cause of the problem is targeted through yoga to deal with the weight problem. It therefore involves detoxification, increasing metabolism, achieving hormonal balance, improving observation & awareness and cardiovascular endurance. Certain forms of yoga prescribe movements done at a rapid pace in a sequential manner that elevates heart rate to moderate or high levels and in such a manner mimic cardiovascular activities. This is very similar to circuit training which is a form of strength training where each muscle group is exercises one after the other without any rest. Such workout principles help in weight loss since heart rate is maintained at a moderate to high level for considerable duration. Apart from the *asanas* that are practiced, *kriyas* such as *kapalbhati* done at a vigorous intensity provides a good cardiovascular endurance workout. Different *asanas* also have different effects on the mind as well. Certain movements performed at a particular pace are known to provide calmness, while other movements help in boosting energy levels. Yoga *asanas* also improve thyroid and pituitary health and balanced secretion of hormones helps in improving metabolism to suit the body's requirements. Other benefits such as reduction in anxiety and detoxification of the body indirectly help in losing weight in a healthy manner. The psychological benefits such as improved awareness and sense of calmness help in immensely improving adherence to weight management program since they bring about a positive attitude towards the entire process.

Meditation for weight management

Meditation refers to the process of reflection and contemplation that helps in calming the mind and in this way relieves stress and anxiety. It has been commonly linked with religion and prayer across many cultures since ancient times. It is often thought of as a tool to improve concentration and as an aid to attaining peace of mind, a path to God and spirituality. Meditation is commonly done by mental exercises that include concentrated breathing, single point focussing as well as chanting. In some cultures it is performed by being completely detached from external worldly contacts while in others the person may interact with the outside world while practicing meditation.

Meditation has developed over centuries and across cultures and civilizations. There is no one form of meditation that fits all the requirements and is ideal for each and everyone practicing it. Which form suits whom depend on factors like state of mind, personality traits and external surroundings. The meditation form that should be practiced is the one in which the person feels most comfortable rather than going after something which is perceived by people in close contact to be most helpful. There is no one single source or authority or text that is referred to for meditation practices. Numerous different forms have evolved over ages each having certain distinct characteristics. A high proportion of these forms though, involve awareness of breath as the underlying platform on which meditation is practiced. Different types of meditation include the following:

1. *Mindfulness meditation* is a popular practice in the West in which awareness of the surroundings is not blocked out. The idea in this practice is to allow all the thoughts to flow into the mind without focusing on any single one of them. This form does not necessarily require quiet and peaceful surroundings and can be performed anywhere. Breathing like most meditation forms is important but is not the primary and sole element. It is a form which is suited to beginners who may find concentrating and blocking out thoughts to focus on nothingness extremely difficult.
2. *Focused meditation* involves focusing on a single thought throughout the practice session. The point of focus can be internal like an imagined object and can also be external in nature like a chant. The emphasis is not on the thought but

on the process of maintaining concentration and not losing focus.

3. *Spiritual meditation* is a form which is closely interlinked with religion and is suited to individuals who offer prayers as part of their daily rituals. The emphasis is on communication and interaction with God and union with the Universal.
4. *Trance based meditation* is an advanced form of spiritual meditation that involves reaching a state of trance by losing self control induced by usage of intoxicating substances. Since the person practicing this form of meditation may not have any memory of the experience, it has a very limited usage, if any, on daily life.
5. *Movement meditation* is a form in which the practice involves constant movement. These movements can be slow & rhythmic in nature such as swaying of the body. These gentle movements are believed to have a calming influence on the mind.
6. *Other forms of meditation* include mantra meditation, transcendental meditation, *kundalini* meditation, *Qi gong* meditation and *Zazen* meditation. Each of them originating in different ages and different parts of the world; differing in the way they are practiced and in terms of their end objectives as well.

Since it is not an exact science, the benefits of meditation cannot be directly and objectively measured. Interest in the scientific community has increased immensely as a result of observations, but studies and research has not determined conclusive proof of benefits derived from meditation. Physical benefits include elimination of stress leading to improvement in conditions such as hypertension and diabetes. The vibrations released are also known to have the added effect of diminishing the negative impact of the disease. Meditation is known to reduce the level of Cortisol and hence reduces stress levels; it also reduces the accumulation of lactic acid which is associated with anxiety. Meditation helps in breath control thereby reducing heart rate and helping the body fight against hypertension; it helps to improve immunity, provides balance to the hormonal system, improves fertility, reduces cholesterol level and helps in weight loss.

While weight loss cannot be directly achieved through meditation it has a more important role to play than any other parameter including physical exercise and diet & nutrition. Meditation does not burn fat in the body but it provides a frame of mind and attitude that is crucial for the efficient functioning of the tools that result in weight loss. Without a positive frame of mind adherence to the weight management program is practically impossible. Meditation helps in identifying the root cause of the weight problem and it does not superficially work on the symptoms of the problem. Even if an individual on a weight loss program is able to achieve weight loss, it may not be sustainable and permanent in case the root cause is not tackled. Meditation helps in improving self control and thereby increases determination that helps in adhering to the program. Moreover, the positive attitude with which the program is adopted magnifies the benefits that may be derived. From the psychological perspective of filling in voids, people have a tendency to go on binges – commonly termed as emotional eating. Meditation helps by working on elimination of desire itself helping the individual practicing it to remain unaffected by the pressures of daily home and work life. The positive attitude that is manifested helps to attain a balance in life. This balance prevents excessive emotions either positive or negative. The person thus practicing experiences an ever prevalent calmness irrespective of the external environment and the alterations that these parameters may undergo. While meditation objectively may not lead to weight loss in the conventional sense, it empowers the individual with a positive attitude – the most useful tool in attaining any weight loss goal.

Meditation also provides numerous psychological benefits. It helps ease stress & anxiety as mentioned earlier. A person becomes calm & composed and is able to visualize the external world with detachment helping in decision making process. Meditation also recharges and provides a feeling of rejuvenation which increases efficiency of all work that the person indulges in. Practicing meditation on a regular basis provides greater mental control that helps in curbing fluctuations in mood and emotion. The spiritual benefits that are derived from regular practice of meditation are manifested in the attitude of kindness and compassion towards others. Union of mind, body and soul leads to an infinite source of love. All these benefits from meditation practice helps produce a balanced personality unfazed by external events and conditions.

Conclusion

For a successful weight management program it is imperative that all these components or pillars be incorporated. When these pillars are not in sync the chances of success of these plans reduces considerably. In fact, neglecting any one of these components may compromise short term as well as long term health and wellness. On the other hand when the wavelengths of the efforts do not match it is very unlikely that the weight management goals are achieved. A positive attitude towards a weight management program that includes a well rounded physical fitness routine, a balanced diet & nutrition plan and sufficient rest & relaxation is almost a guarantee to achieving long term and sustainable weight loss.

Body Weight

What is body weight?

Our Body Weight is the force that the earth exerts on our bodies due to gravitational pull. Everything else remains the same, only the constituent elements in our bodies change causing a change in our body weight. Therefore, let us first understand the composition of the human body.

The human body primarily comprises of water, bones, organs, lean muscle and fat. Within the context of a weight management program, the most important components are lean muscle and fat, since only these can be controlled with proper exercise, diet and nutrition. They can be clubbed together into two basic categories – body fat & fat free weight. Good physical fitness as well as appearance is defined by these two parameters. Low fat percentage in the body and high fat free weight indicate a good body composition.

Body Composition

Body composition analysis refers to the method used to determine the percentage of each of the constituent elements of the body, importantly body fat and lean muscle tissue percentages. There are many methods employed to perform body composition analysis. Traditionally measurement calipers were used to measure the fat in multiple places in the body. This method is cheap and easy to perform but it is not very accurate. Fat itself is of two types – subcutaneous and visceral. Subcutaneous fat is the fat that is present under the skin and is distributed all over the body. Visceral fat is the fat around the organs present for their protection and cushioning. This fat is clearly visible in the abdominal region. The usage of calipers to perform skin fold measurements is based on the principle that fat gets proportionally distributed all over the body. By estimating the total subcutaneous fat, it is possible to determine total body fat percentage.

Hydrostatic weighing is a very accurate method to perform body composition analysis but it is quite cumbersome. Its accuracy is so high that it is sometimes called the gold standard for body composition. It utilizes Archimedes principle to measure body density by immersing the entire body in water. Lean muscle tissue is heavier in comparison to fat, and using the measurement of body density as calculated in hydrostatic weighing it is possible to estimate body fat percentage.

New technologies that are used for body composition analysis include methods such as Bioelectric Impedance Analysis (BIA), Dual Energy X-ray Absorptiometry (DEXA) and Ultrasound. With research & development these methods have now become commercially usable and viable. In common practice, bioelectric impedance analysis and ultrasound are nowadays are commonly used for the purpose. Both BIA and Ultrasound are convenient methods for body composition since they can be performed with high accuracy in a short period of time. Moreover, the equipment used for the purpose is small and portable. BIA uses a small electrical current to flow through the body to calculate electrical resistance. Fat is a bad conductor of electricity. By measuring the magnitude of this resistance or impedance it is possible to estimate fat percentage. Ultrasound uses high frequency sound waves to perform the analysis since the response of fat to ultrasound waves is very different from the response of lean mass in the body. Earlier, body composition analysis was used sparingly for technical studies and research. However, with the requirement posed by the burgeoning fitness and wellness industry, it is now commonly used. There are many advantages of performing body composition analysis on a regular basis.

- ✓ It helps in determining the health status of the member by calculating the fat mass and lean muscle mass. Greater the lean muscle mass healthier is the individual. Lesser the fat mass healthier is the individual.
- ✓ It helps the exercise programmer in designing the exercise card and the nutrition counselor to prepare a diet plan on the basis of the analysis. The target of fitness programs is to increase lean muscle tissue and decrease fat percentage.
- ✓ Body composition analysis done on a regular basis helps in determining the progress of a weight management program. Changes can be introduced in the program after analyzing the effects of the previous exercise program and diet plan on the body composition.

A typical body composition analysis provides a lot of information and measures numerous different parameters. The parameters that are most important to analyze include the following:

1. **Weight** – It is the total body weight in kilograms or pounds.
2. **Skeletal Muscle Mass (SMM)** – It is the total weight of lean muscle tissue in the body expressed in kilograms or pounds.
3. **Body Fat Mass** – It is the total fat mass measured in kilograms or pounds. It includes both the subcutaneous fat and visceral fat
4. **Fat Free Mass** – It is the total weight of the non-fat part of the body. (Fat Free Mass = Weight – Body Fat Mass). It is measured in kilograms or pounds.
5. **Body Mass Index (BMI)** – It is a value which is used to classify whether the person is obese, overweight, underweight or normal. It is commonly used as the parameter when body composition analyzers are not available. It is like a thumb rule and tells us with a simple arithmetic calculation, as to which category a person belongs to. *BMI = (Weight in Kilograms)/(Height in meters)*^{2}. BMI works well in most cases however, it only takes into consideration body weight (height of a person is assumed to be constant after adulthood). BMI calculations will classify a body builder as obese, since the body weight will be higher despite most of it being lean muscle and not fat. In such cases where distinction between fat and lean mass is important, BMI does not provide the correct results. It is therefore imperative to measure body fat and lean muscle percentages separately.
6. **Percentage Body Fat** – It is the body fat mass expressed as a percentage of body weight. Percentage Body Fat = {(Body Fat Mass)/(Weight)}*100. This is the most useful as well as important parameter that is used while designing a weight management program. In general, males have a body fat percentage in the range of 10 to 20%. In females due to the sex hormone estrogen, body fat percentage is higher in the range of 20 to 30%.

7. **Resting Metabolic Rate (RMR)** – It is the calories that the body burns in a complete state of rest in a day for essential processes such as respiration and digestion. Greater the lean muscle mass in the body greater will be the BMR, and hence the body will be able to burn more number of calories throughout the day.

The Body Composition analysis also gives a segmental analysis of the fat mass and lean muscle tissue in the body. It calculates the mass of fat and lean muscle in the left arm, right arm, left leg, right leg and trunk. This information may be utilized in case there are fitness goals that are specifically related to increase in lean muscle and consequently weight gain. Segmental analysis may not be too useful for weight loss, since the aim is to reduce the body fat percentage. As fat is present throughout the body, the proportion in which fat loss happens is commensurate to this distribution. Contrary to popular myth, spot reduction of fat cannot take place since fat is an energy substrate that will reduce when it is used for metabolism for production of energy that the body requires.

Overweight & Obesity

The weight of an individual should be within a particular prescribed range. This range typically measured as percentage of body fat depends on parameters such as age, sex, height etc. When the fat percentage in the body is above the prescribed range, the person is said to be overweight. A certain basic amount of fat is required in the body for essential functions such as protection of organs and temperature regulation, but when the percentage goes beyond the range then it starts having detrimental effects on the body. When the percentage of body fat goes even higher, the individual is said to be obese. Obesity is one of the most common lifestyle diseases plaguing the world population. Over a billion people in the world are either overweight or are obese and more than 60% of the adult population in Unite States of America falls under this classification. Despite the level of awareness going up on a continuous basis, the prevalence of obesity has been on the rise over the past many years. Obesity puts the individual at high risk to numerous health issues such as coronary and cardiovascular disease, diabetes and other chronic ailments thereby drastically reducing life expectancy. In the ages gone by being overweight or obese was considered to be a sign of wealth over the years there has been a cultural swing with people now understanding the issues associated with being overweight and obese. It is also manifested in the fact that being overweight or obese is not considered physically appealing any more, and being slim and looking fit is far more preferable.

A common quick thumb rule that can be used for determining whether a person is overweight or obese is Body Mass Index. In case the BMI of a person is more than 25 the person is classified as being overweight while in case it goes above 30, the person is said to be obese. There are various degrees or levels of obesity – level 1 to 3 and specifies the extent of obesity in the individual with a BMI which is greater than 40 is classified as morbid obesity. The exact number range is defined by World Health Organization but other health bodies have made certain modification to suit specific populations since ethnicity also has a role to play in the way obesity is classified as well as the way in which the problem is approached. For example, the negative impact of excess fat percentage is greater at lower levels of BMI in case of Asian population in comparison to Caucasians. As a result of this, in Asian countries, the range for classification as obese starts at 25 itself. As mentioned earlier as well, it is important to understand that BMI is only an indicator and may not be accurate in specific cases such as when body weight is high but lean muscle tissue is greater and fat percentage is pretty low. In terms of body fat percentage, the normal range is 20 to 30% for females and 10 to 20% among males. A person is said to be obese when the fat percentage in the body goes above the upper limit of the range. Body fat percentage is a more accurate indicator, but BMI is in common practice because of ease of measurement and calculation.

Spread of obesity

Overweight and Obesity expose the individual to numerous risk factors, and is now globally considered fifth in the list of risks leading to death. According to WHO around 3 million people die each year through indirect effects of being overweight or obese. There are more than 1.6 billion adults who are overweight with around 10% of the global population classified in the obese category. The distribution in terms of sex is more or less even with the around 40% of the obese category being males 60% of the category as females. The problem exists even with children; for children under the age of five, close to 45 million lie in the overweight category with more than 80% of these children living in under–developed and developing countries of the world.

In the United States of America, according to NHANES, 33% of adults (over the age of 20 years) are overweight, 35.7% are classified as being obese and 6.3% in the morbid obesity category. Since the late 1980s there has been a steady increase in percentage of the adult population in the obese category, rising from around 23% in 1988 to more than 36% as on date. In the last decade, this percentage of obese women has remained more or less the same, while it has steadily increased in a linear fashion for men. During the period from 1980 to 2010, while the percentage of obese people more than doubled, the percentage of people in the overweight category more or less remained the same.

There is no significant variation in the change in percentage of obese males within various ethnic groups. For non-Hispanic white men, the percentage jumped from 20.3% in 1988 to 36.2% in 2012; for non-Hispanic black men, it jumped from 21.1% in 1988 to 38.8% in 2012; for Mexican- American men, it jumped from 23.9% in 1988 to 36.6% in 2012. As can be observed there is no significant variation in case of males. However, in case of females a stark difference is seen for non-Hispanic black women. For non-Hispanic white women, the percentage jumped from 22.9% in 1988 to 32.2% in 2012; for non-Hispanic black women, it jumped from 38.4% in 1988 to 58.5% in 2012; for Mexican- American women, it jumped from 35.4% in 1988 to 44.9% in 2012.

Obesity in children also called childhood obesity is also posing a significant global problem. Steadily but surely the percentage of children who are overweight and obese has gone up attaining significant proportions. In the United States of America, according to a NHANES study conducted in 2009-10, 16.9% of all children in the age group 2 to 19 were obese. If we look at the break-up, for children in the age group 2 to 5 years, the percentage of obese children increased from 5% in 1980 to 12.1% in 2010; for children in the age category 6 to 11, this percentage increased from 6.5% in 1980 to 18.0% in 2010; for children in the age category 12 to 19 this percentage increased from 5% in 1980 to 18.4% in 2010. If we study the last decade in isolation, for boys there was a significant increase in percentage who were obese, but it remained more or less the same in case of girls.

The number of older adults, defined as people over the age of 65 in the United States of America is expected to double by the year 2050. In terms of numbers, the expected increase is from around 43 million to about 88 million. This increase is due to a combination of an increase in population and the availability of better and more advanced medical facilities and services thereby improving life expectancy. Around 35% of people in the older adult category were obese in 2010. This corresponded to 8 million in the age group 65 to 74, roughly 40.8% of this category and about 5 million in the age group 75 and above, which is approximately 27.8% of the category. Over the last decade the percentage of obese males in the 65 to 74 age category has gone up from 31.6% in 2000 to 41.5% in 2010. For the above 75 age group category the increase was from 17.7% in 2000 to 26.5% in 2010. During this duration, the change in percentages among females was not significant.

In terms of ethnic background, the observation was contrary to the above case. The difference in males of this age group was not so significant. However, among women – in the age group 65 to 74 years, 53.9% of non-Hispanic black women were obese, 38.9 % of non-Hispanic white women and 46.6% for Hispanic women. In the age group 75 years and above, 49.4% of non-Hispanic black women were obese, 27.5% of non-Hispanic white women and 30.2% for Hispanic women. As can be seen ethnic differences translated into genetic as well as social & cultural reasons has significant impact on obesity levels.

Effects of obesity on health

Obesity is called the silent killer. It may not directly lead to death in the manner other disease do, but it indirectly leads to numerous chronic ailments and issues that reduce life expectancy. It is one of the most preventable reasons for death. It has been established in numerous studies that people with low BMI levels are at a lower mortality risk in comparison to those with higher BMI. In the United States alone, about half a million deaths occur every year due to obesity related issues. On an average life expectancy goes down by around two years in case a person is overweight and up to ten years in case of morbid obesity.

Obesity is known to increase the risk of numerous physical, mental and emotional problems. In some cases obesity is directly responsible for manifestation of these chronic ailments, while in others, the correlation is strong because of common causes such as inadequate physical activity, poor diet & nutritional habits and overall sedentary lifestyle. In general, the diseases correlated with obesity can be classified into two basic categories – diseases that occur due to an increase in fat mass and disease that occur due to increase in the number of fat cells in the body. The first category includes osteoarthritis, social isolation and sleep apnea, while the second category includes diseases such as cardiovascular diseases, cancer and diabetes. The most common ailments that are associated with or are correlated with obesity areas following:

1. Type 2 Diabetes - More than 80% of type 2 diabetes patients are overweight or obese. This correlation occurs in men and women alike. This form of diabetes arises when the pancreas stops producing adequate amount of insulin or the cells in the body are not able to utilize the insulin that has been secreted by the pancreas. Whenever there is an increase in sugar level in the blood, pancreas secretes the hormone insulin to help in its metabolism. Obesity severely limits the capacity of insulin to control blood sugar level. As a result of this the body starts to secrete more and more insulin to keep up with the increased blood sugar level, but in the end it is not able to keep the level in range any longer.
2. Cardiovascular & Neurological diseases – Obese people are at high risk to cardiovascular and heart diseases such as myocardial ischemia or heart attack, angina pectoris, con-

gestive heart failure and arrhythmia. This is because they are prone to increased LDL Cholesterol and triglyceride levels in the blood along with their tendency to develop hypertension or high blood pressure. These are the main ingredients that lead to coronary and cardiovascular diseases. Heart attacks are caused by blockages created in the artery that provides oxygen to the myocardial muscles. These symptoms also lead to stroke which occurs when inadequate amount of oxygen reaches the brain. Excess visceral fat or the fat in the abdominal region leads to blood vessels getting inflamed which further raise the risk of these diseases. In the United States coronary artery disease and stroke are the leading causes of death.

3. Hypertension – The blood flowing in the arteries exerts pressure on the arterial wall. This pressure is measured as the blood pressure. Obesity has a direct correlation with blood pressure levels. Individuals already having high blood pressure can see dramatic decrease in the blood pressure levels by decreasing body weight.
4. Metabolic syndrome – It is a group of disorders that which when occur together increase drastically the risk of developing cardiovascular diseases as well as diabetes. These factors include android or central obesity, increased blood pressure, increased blood sugar level, reduced HDL Cholesterol level and increased triglyceride level in the blood. Metabolic syndrome is one of the biggest obesity related issues in the country. Almost 22% of the adult population suffers from metabolic syndrome, in terms of numbers it translates to more than 50 million people.
5. Polycystic Ovary syndrome – It is one of the most common issues faced by women of reproductive age. A majority of these women are overweight and obese. In this syndrome underdeveloped follicles get accumulated in the ovaries leading to menstrual cycles being irregular, above normal hair growth and ovarian cysts. It leads to insulin resistance putting women with this problem at a risk of developing dia-

betes at a later stage. Even in adolescent girls, high insulin level in the blood, resistance to insulin and obesity are all related to PCOS.

6. Dyslipidemia - It is the condition in which the lipid profile of the blood becomes adverse – HDL cholesterol or the good cholesterol goes down, while triglyceride and LDL cholesterol or the bad cholesterol increases. This is often a result of increase in weight and results in coronary artery disease. Losing weight has a direct correlation with improvement in lipid profile.
7. Gastrointestinal problems
    a. Cholelithiasis – Commonly called gallstones happens when high cholesterol content leads to hardening of bile. These hard, rock like pieces cause severe back and abdominal back pain. In some cases even surgical intervention may be required to remove the gall stones.
    b. GERD or Gastroesophageal reflex disease – It is a disease in which the muscles at the bottom of the esophagus allows the stomach contents along with other digestive juices to enter the esophagus
    c. Fatty Liver Disease – In this disease fat builds up in the liver leading to inflammation and damages the liver severely by forming fibrous tissues. In some severe cases it can lead to irreversible liver damage as well as liver cirrhosis.
    d. Colon cancer – This kind of cancer leads to cancerous kind of growth in the colon, appendix and the rectum.
    e. Hernia – The contents of certain body cavities bulge out from their normal areas in hernia. The content includes fatty tissue enclosed in very thin layers or membranes
8. Genitourinary problems
    a. Erectile dysfunction is the inability to maintain an erection of the penis in order for sexual intercourse

b. Renal failure – This is chronic in nature when the kidneys fail to perform their main function – excreting waste material from the body.

c. Incontinence – Reduced bladder control leading to slight amount of leakage of urine and also to uncontrolled wetting in severe cases

d. Hypogonadism – The hormonal production of the sex organs of the body become greatly diminished or my stop completely

e. Other such problems include uterine and breast cancer, which refers to cancerous growth in the uterus and breast

9. Respiratory problems

a. Sleep Apnea – The person suffering from this disorder experiences repeated pauses in breathing during sleep. This may occur multiple times and may last for many breaths.

f. Hypoventilation syndrome – The person facing this disorder does not get enough oxygen during sleep. This results in high carbon dioxide levels in the blood and consequently low oxygen levels.

g. Dyspnea – This refers to the gamut of disorders that result in shortness of breath manifested by extreme difficulty in breathing

10. Musculoskeletal problems

a. Osteoarthritis – It is a disease that affects the joints of the body, commonly the knees, lower back and hips. It occurs due to wearing away of the protective cartilage around the joints. Due to obesity there is extra load on these weight carrying joints and the extent of the disorder aggravates further.

11. Psychological problems
    a. Depression – An obese individual may undergo severe bouts of depression wherein there may be a perennial feeling of sadness and hopelessness.
    h. Diminished self confidence - People who are obese and due to various reasons have not been successful in reducing their weight may have extremely low self esteem and low self confidence and this feeling gets stronger as once fails repeatedly in the effort.

Causes of obesity

Obesity in general is caused by an excess intake of energy through a combination of improper diet and inadequate physical activity. There may however, also be contributing elements such as genetics, medical conditions and disorders. However, this lack of energy balance is the underlying reason behind weight gain. This happens when energy input in the form of food provides more energy than that is expended as energy output by the body. Energy output is a combination of a number of factors.

1. Resting Metabolic Rate (RMR) – It is the total number of calories that the body is able to burn at a state of rest in a day for essential activities of daily life such as respiration, digestion etc.
2. Cost of Activity (COA) – It refers to the total calories that an individual may burn in a day owing to his or her activities of daily life. These include energy burnt during work. Therefore, a person working an office may burn only 300 calories in an entire working day, while a person who is a supervisor of a real estate firm on the field, will burn at least 600 calories is a day.
3. Cost of Exercise (COE) – It is the calories that a person burns while participating in physical activities such as walking, jogging, swimming and exercising in a gym. This will include energy burnt doing cardiovascular endurance workouts as well resistance training workouts.

4. Thermic Effect of Food (TEF) – Our body requires some energy for breaking down food to release energy. However, some foods such as glucose are absorbed easily while complex compounds like protein require energy to break down and be utilized. Therefore, what is consumed plays an essential role in calculation of Thermic effect of Food.
5. Other factors – Certain other parameters play a very minor role. For example, adaptive thermogenesis is the regulation of heat production in the body as a result of changes in the external environment, this leads to greater inefficiency in metabolism. Shivering in the cold is a distinct example of adaptive thermogenesis. For all practical purposes the magnitude of this is very small and we do not take it into consideration for calculation of energy output.

The net sum of all these parameters is energy output. The total energy released as a result of metabolism of food that has been ingested is energy input. Our diet is a combination of energy compounds that release energy during metabolism; it also should include micronutrients such as vitamins & minerals that are required in small quantities to act as catalysts in various biochemical reactions in the body; finally water and fiber also play an important role in our body and should be consumed in adequate quantities. However, for calculation of energy input we consider the energy released from the breakdown of energy compounds that are consumed as part of the weight management diet plan.

1. 1 gram of carbohydrate releases 4 calories of energy
2. 1 gram of protein releases 4 calories of energy
3. 1 gram of fat releases 9 calories of energy
4. 1 gram of alcohol releases 7 calories of energy

A simple arithmetic exercise will tell us the net calorie intake during the day – this is essentially the energy input component. When energy output is less than energy input then there is energy excess in the body. As can be expected, the body stores this excess energy in the body for utilization during times when there may not be enough energy input to the body. This is the primary cause of weight gain and there are numerous reasons as to why this energy input is greater than energy output that creates this imbalance that leads to weight gain.

Diet

When energy input is more than energy output, weight gain results. Energy input is nothing but the food we ingest. When we eat more food that releases more energy than what we require, it gets stored in the body. Some part of this excess is stored in the form of glycogen in the liver and muscles, but after this it is predominantly stored as fat. This results in a person being overweight initially which then translates in to obesity in case the situation is not controlled. Over the last two decades it has been seen that the increase in percentage of obese people in the adult population of United States has been matched by an increase in the average calorie intake per capita per day. The increase in women was around 350 calories per day while that for men was 170 calories per day. All this extra energy being consumed comes primarily from simple carbohydrates from junk and convenience foods. Consumption of refined high fat food along with sweetened beverages is the primary contributors of this increase in calories per day. The dependence of the average population on these easily available convenience products has increased considerably.

Sedentary Lifestyle

Over the years there has been a big shift away from work that is physically demanding. With the mechanization of almost all kinds of physical work, working hours of most individuals involve hardly any physical labor. For example, in agricultural practices, the demand for physical labor which was quite significant has drastically come down with advent of machines that complete all jobs from harvesting to threshing by the press of a few buttons. In addition, the propensity towards leisure activities that provide no physical exercise whatsoever, such playing computer games. Children as well as adults no longer indulge in recreation activities, and even if they do, physically challenging activities are not preferred. In children this lack of adequate physical activity is leading to an increased incidence in the cases of childhood obesity. It is one of the rapidly growing problems of American society and needs to be addressed soon, since childhood obesity translates into various ailments and disorders at a very early stage in life. Consequently, both life expectancy and quality of life diminish rapidly. Sedentary lifestyle has in this manner reduced the energy output component of the equation leading to the imbalance that causes obesity.

Genetics

The link between genetics and obesity has been well researched and documented. Studies have shown that genes have a significant contribution towards weight gain, in both direct as well as indirect ways. Genes have a direct effect on hormonal secretion, insulin resistance, metabolic rate etc. These parameters have an important contribution in the energy balance equation. Indirectly, genes have a significant influence on habits and lifestyle pattern which leads to choices being made that eventually effect the energy balance equation. Studies that have been done on inheritance patterns have concluded that the offspring of two obese people will in more than 75% of the cases be obese. In stark contrast this figure is only 10% in case both the parents have normal weight. Genes also play a significant role in determining where in the body, the extra fat will be stored. A study of body shapes revealed that there is significant correlation between body type and shape of parent and offspring.

Medical Conditions

Numerous medical conditions and disorders lead to the individual being overweight and obese. Hypothyroidism or low activity level of thyroid gland results in low levels of secretion of the thyroid hormone which is essentially a growth hormone. This has a significant influence on the metabolic rate of the body. When insufficient hormone is released it leads to low metabolic rate and consequently the person feels extremely weak. Even after a complete night's sleep the person gets up in a partial state of fatigue. Lethargy and sluggishness is experienced throughout the day. All these factors especially low metabolic rate contribute in weight gain. Polycystic ovarian syndrome or PCOS is a common occurrence in women of reproductive age. Women with PCOS face problems of excessive hair growth and other reproductive issues along with the problem of weight gain. Another example is Cushing's syndrome in which excess cortisone hormone is secreted by the adrenal glands of the body. People with this syndrome gain weight rapidly and tend to store a lot of fat in the upper body typically abdomen, face and neck while still having thin limbs. This syndrome may develop in case high doses of medication such as prednisone are consumed over a period of time. The risk of obesity is seen to be higher in patients with one or the other psychiatric disorders. Numerous medications are also known to cause significant gains in weight. These include antidepressants, antipsychotics, hormones such as insulin, anticonvulsants and some hormonal contraception.

Social causes

Societal changes over the last few generations have in general been responsible directly and indirectly in increasing the spread of obesity. Culturally being obese and overweight was seen as a sign of great wealth. With the understanding of the correlation of obesity with numerous ailments and diseases a significant cultural shift has taken place against obesity. A shift in attraction has taken place from a well rounded body to one which is slim and physically fit. Such a body is considered appealing and desired by most people, this is due to a change in outlook of the society at large.

Inequities presented by social classes have been posited as an important factor in the increase in obesity in both developed and developing nations of the world. In developed societies, people with wealth are in a position to afford nutritious food and are at leisure to choose activities that involve physical fitness. On the other hand in developing as well as under-developed countries of the world, lack of money forcing purchase of high energy foods, lack of leisure time because of survival pressure and general attitude towards body shape, mass and appearance has lead to a rapid increase in obesity levels.

Other reasons

A study conducted a few years back listed a set of various reasons that cause obesity other than the commonly known and accepted ones. These include emotional factors such as stress, anxiety and boredom which may lead to an individual eating without being hungry; late pregnancies that may lead to childhood obesity in the child; women finding it difficult to lose weight that has been gained to support the baby during pregnancy; environmental pollutants such as endocrine disruptors that hamper lipid metabolism in the body; with the advancement of age, there is significant loss of lean muscle mass leading to a reduction in metabolism leading to weight gain; insufficient sleep results in an imbalance in the secretion of hormones *ghrelin* (lack of sleep leads to an increase in this hormone which increases hunger), *leptin* (inadequate sleep leads to a decrease in this hormone which gives a feeling of fullness) and insulin (regulates blood sugar level) that leads to weight gain; other genetic factors that are passed on through generations. There may not be conclusive evidence that these factors are responsible for obesity, but empirical studies provide a reasonably high correlation factor between the cause and the effect.

Weight Management

Weight management refers to the group of activities that are performed to gain weight, lose weight or even maintain it at the same level. As described in the previous sections, the goal of weight management programs is to increase lean muscle tissue in case weight gain is desired and to lose fat in case weight loss in the goal. Any weight management program that causes weight alterations to happen in any other manner compromises health to a certain degree. For example, crash dieting is a common practice for losing weight rapidly. This technique involves going on very low calorie diets making the body burn energy reserves from within rather than depending on resources from food that is eaten. Such a weight management plan will definitely lead to weight loss, but this loss of weight will not be healthy. There will be some loss of fat from the body but the body will lose considerable amount of lean muscle tissue as well. Also, the rate at which weight loss happens should be taken into consideration. A benchmark for healthy weight loss or weight gain is 1 to 2 pounds per week. This will ensure that the body does not have to undergo sudden drastic changes. The effect of weight loss is not just manifested in physical appearances but there are quite a few changes that occur within the body, such as changes in metabolic rate which is directly controlled by the hormonal system. These sudden changes therefore should be avoided for healthy weight loss. Another example is the usage of equipment such as sauna belts. These fancy gadgets became very popular in a very short period of time. The sales campaigns projected the product as a messiah in the fight for weight loss. Since it promised immediate weight loss and showed results to back up the claim, people started using it on a regular basis. The usage of these belts not only leads to weight loss but also to inch loss in specific areas of the body where it is used, such as thighs and abdomen. However, the story is quite different when we take a closer look at it. These belts work by increasing temperature and thereby causing perspiration. This loss of water from the body is what is manifested as weight loss and specifically inch loss. Water is one of the most important constituent elements in the body and makes up a high percentage of our blood. It is responsible for transport of oxygen, nutrients, hormones etc. to and from different parts of the body. The effects of dehydration have been well documented and even experienced by each and every one of us. The call of thirst is a sign that the body is on its way to dehydration. Severe dehydration can also lead to death. In such a perspective, it is apparent that the weight loss caused by dehydration can in no way be deemed healthy at all. Thus, although such products give desired results but the ways in which these results are achieved jeopardize health and safety.

A weight management program can never be a product, in the basic sense that it has to be different for each and every individual. The body composition as well as genetic makeup of each and every one of us is different and so each and every program to alter it will also be different. A program can only be effective as well as healthy when it is customized or tailored for the individual to meet the body's specific requirements. In fact, if all measurable parameters such as body composition remain the same, still the response of one individual versus another to exactly the same program will be different. It is therefore imperative that a weight management program be designed, implemented and manipulated taking into consideration the unique requirements and responses of the individual to it.

Components of Weight Management Program

A healthy weight management program aims to achieve and subsequently maintain optimal body weight. This is done by making healthy lifestyle choices such as participating in a regular physical fitness program, eating a nutritious and balanced diet and taking adequate amount of rest during the day. Each of these components is important in the success of the weight management program. In some cases, a person may not be in a position to make the necessary lifestyle changes that are essential for weigh management. For such cases, medication and surgical treatments are available for the treatment of the problem.

Goal Setting

It is extremely important that the first step in any weight management program be taken with utmost care. Goals should be realistic in nature and at the same time it should be ensured that goals do not compromise health in any manner. The following points should be taken into consideration while setting goals.

1. Adults seeking to lose weight should aim to keep the rate of loss of body weight to 1 to 2 pounds per week. Firstly, this weight loss should happen through loss of body fat and not through loss of lean muscle tissue or water. In case a person loses more weight than this, there are good chances that the loss is happening through the unwanted routes. In any case, regular body composition would provide the true nature of the results and adequate intervention in the weight management program can be introduced after analyzing the results. Secondly, gradual weight loss is imperative since a number of hormonal changes follow weight loss and it is important to give the body time to adjust accordingly.

2. Along with 1 to 2 pound per week thumb rule adults should set goals in the range of loss of 5 to 10% of body weight over a 6 month period. This is a healthy rate and lowers the risk of cardiovascular and coronary artery diseases considerably. After a stabilization period fol-

lowing loss of 10% of body weight, in case the individual is still overweight, further weight loss can be planned.

3. In case of children, the focus should be on getting the child involved in physical activities of one form or the other. The child should also be encouraged to eat healthier. Forcing weight loss goals and making the program objective is not suggested in case of children. In case there is an underlying medical condition that may be the reason for the child being overweight or obese, the involvement of a specialist in the field is often beneficial.

Diet regulation

By regulating the energy intake as part of the weight management program, it is possible to create the energy deficit that is required for weight loss to take place. For burning 1 pound of fat, a deficit of 3,500 calories needs to be created. This means that the difference between energy input and energy output should be 3,500 calories. This will roughly translate into 500 calories per day. Therefore, if the total energy output is 2,000 calories, then the input should be planned in such a manner that the intake does not exceed 1,500 calories. Other important points that should be taken into consideration while preparing a weight management meal plan include:

1. In general, for most women a diet plan providing 1,200 calorie and for most men a plan providing 1,500 calories is sufficient to cause healthy weight loss. In case the individual feels very hungry while following such a weight management plan, then an increase of about 200 calories can be done and then gradually this can be brought back down to calculated levels.
2. Very low calorie diets and crash dieting should not be indulged in. Apart from the loss of lean muscle tissue in the body, it may even lead to an increase of fat storage in the body. Since fat is an energy dense molecule, the body will go into starvation mode and try and conserve fat at the expense of lean muscle which is difficult to maintain. Further,

these low calorie diets may cause other health issues due to lack of proper nutrition being provided for the body.

3. For children and teenagers, the calorie content of food should not be too low. The emphasis should be on eating healthy. In case calorie content of the meals goes below a certain level, it starts hampering the growth of the body which is absolutely undesirable.

4. A balanced and nutritious diet should never be compromised upon. All the macro and micro nutrients have a specific role to play in the proper functioning of the body and the absence or deficiency of even one of these nutrients may lead to medical disorders and consequently be detrimental to overall health. In general, the nutrients can be segregated into 3 categories. The first category includes energy compounds that provide energy to the body when they undergo metabolism – carbohydrates, proteins and fats. The second category includes micro nutrients that are required in small quantities to act as catalysts in various biochemical reactions of the body – vitamins & minerals. The third category includes water & fiber which apart from helping in the digestion of food play other important roles in the body as well. The following points need to be considered while preparing a weight loss meal plan for an individual looking to lose weight.

    a. The diet should be balanced in such a manner that all the nutrients are made available in adequate quantities for the optimal functioning of the body. For micro nutrients, a reference index such as Daily Value (DV) or Recommended Dietary Allowance (RDA) can be used for calculating the amounts in which all these nutrients should be consumed.

    b. The variation in the quantities of energy compounds – carbohydrates, fats and proteins depends on the fitness goals of the individual. Specifically, the quantities are dependent upon whether the person wants to gain or lose weight and also on the rate at which this is desired. In general, 50 to 60% of the energy requirement of the body should be met from carbohydrates, around 20 to 30% from fats and 15 to 20% from proteins. Apart from providing energy, these macro nutrients have other important roles to play in the body and therefore presence in these adequate quantities is deemed imperative.

c. Water should be consumed in adequate quantities. 2 to 3 liters per day is a good amount. This may however vary depending on the environment and parameters such as altitude, humidity and temperature. Fiber is important for digestion and proper amounts should be ingested. 25 to 35 grams of fiber per day is meets the daily requirements of the body.

d. The body requires energy at a particular rate. In case more energy is available at a particular point in time than what it can utilize it starts storing this energy in the form of fat. This is the primary reason why heavy meals should be avoided. Instead, an individual looking to lose weight should go in for low calorie high frequency meals. Following a 6 meal plan ensures that the body is provided enough nourishment, at the same time it does not convert and store the extra energy as fat.

e. Foods that need to be avoided include simple carbohydrates such as sucrose or sugar and glucose which release energy instantly and in case the body does not require the energy it converts the excess and stores it in the form of body fat. Foods rich in trans-fat, saturated fat and cholesterol should be avoided since taking them in large quantities lead to cardiovascular and coronary artery diseases. These include red meat, meat of organs such as liver, dairy products which are high in fat content such as cream and butter, coconut and palm oil, food such as fries cooked in partially hydrogenated oils, egg yolk, and shrimp.

f. Food that can be used as substitutes include canola oil, olive oil, low fat dairy products, lean protein sources such as fish and chicken breast, whole grain foods and plenty of vegetables & fruits.

Physical activity

Physical activity will increase the energy output that is achieved on a daily basis and help create an energy deficit. This energy deficit will ultimately help in losing weight. Apart from this primary benefit other benefits of regular physical activity include the following:

1. Regular cardiovascular endurance workout helps in improving the efficiency of the cardiovascular system which is responsible for oxygen delivery and utilization in working muscles of the body. It also improves the functioning of the heart leading to chronic adaptations such as lowering of resting heart rate. The functioning of lungs is also positively affected by regular cardiovascular activity.
2. It helps in reduction of risks of cardiovascular disease, coronary artery disease, diabetes, hypertension and cancers
3. Resistance training helps in increasing the lean muscle tissue in the body and also helps in strengthening the joints. Since form of bones follow functionality, resistance training imparts enough stimulus on the bones to strengthen them and also reduce the rate at which loss of bone mineral density occurs.
4. Flexibility training helps improve the range of motion about the joints and prevents injuries that seem to occur fairly commonly in individuals with poor flexibility.
5. Regular exercise helps in improving quality of sleep and also helps the mind to cope with stressful conditions in a better manner.

The major components of an exercise program include muscular strength, muscular endurance, cardiovascular endurance and flexibility. Whatever the goals of the exercise program may be, it is imperative to include all these components of exercise in a program for optimal fitness. In general, a balanced workout program for weight loss should include 30 to 40 minutes of cardiovascular aerobic activity for at least 3 times a week such that heart rate is at moderate levels, resistance training for 2 to 3 times in a week for all major muscle groups such that each group is covered at least once during the week and flexibility training in the form of static stretching for at least 2 to 3 times in a week. The program should be such that the intensity is not increased beyond the comfort level of the participant until and unless all the techniques of exercise are properly learnt. The intensity of the program should increase gradually and can be achieved through progressive overloading leading to improved results. Children should participate in different activities for at least an hour on a daily basis. This should predominantly be aerobic in nature and can include a variety of exercises. However, resistance training with heavy weights should be avoided completely, since this may hamper the growth process of the bones.

Behavioral changes

To achieve success in weight management programs it is important to introduce behavioral changes to make it conducive for the participant to adhere to the program. The following steps can help immensely in this process:

1. A change in surroundings plays a big role in improving adherence to the program. Simple steps include avoiding eating in front of the television; this leads to overeating since the person is not generally concentrating on what is being eaten. A change of clothes can be carried to work in case exercise is possible close to the workplace, since coming back home after work and then going out to exercise again may be difficult to do. Instead of unhealthy snacks being readily available all around the house, it is better to substitute these with health snacks and salads, so that even if hunger pangs are experienced and food is eaten against the plan, only healthy options are available for consumption.
2. It is important to keep a log while following a weight management plan both for diet as well as for exercise. This helps in understanding what works and what does not work well

within the program. Also, it helps in analyzing the program results objectively.

3. It is important to consult experts in the field of nutrition as well as exercise physiology, especially in case there is an underlying medical condition which may have resulted in weight gain. Also, in case of any contraindications, exercise should be avoided and it should in no case be performed without the consent of a health specialist.
4. A reward system should be part of any weight management program, since it helps in creating the right environment and motivates the person to adhere to the program.

Medication

In certain cases when lifestyle changes may not be possible to incorporate, such as when due to an underlying medical condition, a person may not be able to perform physical exercise or when a person is morbidly obese and cannot even walk properly, medication for weight loss may be prescribed. A few FDA approved drugs that are used for weight loss include the following:

1. Orlistat can be used to lose weight in the range of around 5 to 10 pounds; however some people may be able to lose more than that. It is most effective in the first 6 months of drug usage. It should be consumed only under prescription from a physician who will need to monitor the progress as well as track any side effects that be experienced as a result of usage of the drug. It works by reducing the absorption of fats and fat soluble vitamins A, D, E and K. Side effects include loose stools. Liver damage may also occur in some cases. It should also be avoided in case blood thinning medication is being consumed for treatment of thyroid diseases and diabetes.
2. Lorcaserin Hydrochloride can be used for weight loss for adults with BMI over 30. The consumption of the drug should be accompanied by proper dietary regulation as well as regular physical exercise. It is generally prescribed for people who have a maximum of one obesity related medical condition or disorder such as diabetes or hypertension.

3. There are certain medicines that are not FDA approved but are known to be used in the treatment of severe and morbid obesity. These include anti-depressants, medication used to treat seizures such as zonisamide and topiramate and medicines used to treat diabetes such as metformin.
    a. Certain OTC products which are not FDA approved because they are sold as dietary supplements rather than medication are utilized for achieving weight loss. These include products such as:
    b. Chromium - It is an element that is used for weight loss, but correlation is not clearly established. Moreover, there are serious side effects that come along with the usage of chromium.
    c. Ephedra or *ma huang* - Ephedra derived from plants contains *ephedrine* which is its active ingredient. It can lead to short term weight loss but has severe long term side effects such as increased blood pressure levels.
    d. *Hoodia* cactus found in Africa is used as an appetite suppressant, and its effectiveness and safety are not known.
    e. Diuretics and laxatives are commonly used for weight loss, but the weight lost is due to reduction in water and not in fat. Consumption can lead to loss of potassium in the blood and can lead to heart and muscle problems in the long run.

Surgical Procedures

In cases of morbid obesity i.e. with people having a BMI of more than 40, surgical procedures may be suggested. It may also be applicable for people with BMI greater than 35 but with a life threatening condition such as severe type 2 diabetes, cardiomyopathy and sleep apnea. Weight loss surgeries can be classified into two categories:

1. Gastroplasty – It involves using a band or even staples to create a small bag or pouch in the top section of the stomach.

This essentially reduces the amount of food that the stomach is capable of holding.

2. Gastric bypass – It involves creating a bypass around a part of small intestine which is responsible for absorption of the calories. This form of surgery limits the intake of food and limits the number of calories that are absorbed by the body. There are a few side effects such as diarrhea, light headedness and nausea.

Surgeries are effective in the long run only when they are followed up with regular physical activity and balanced diet as part of a weight management program, once the weight has been brought down to manageable levels.

Weight Management – Maintenance phase

It is one thing to lose the excess weight and another to actually maintain the new weight. For a number of people, after weight goals are achieved, relapse is quite a common occurrence and people tend to gain back all the lost weight. It is therefore extremely important to consider a weight management program as a new lifestyle rather than an object oriented short term intervention. Consuming a balanced and nutritious diet, regular physical workout and proper rest & relaxation should be incorporated and accepted as part of the new lifestyle; these have been taken up as permanent features of life, and should be enjoyed and cherished.

Body goals diary

Body goals diary

Body goals diary

Body goals diary

Body goals diary

Body goals diary

Body goals diary

Body goals diary

Body goals diary

Body goals diary

Body goals diary

Body goals diary

Body goals diary

Body goals diary

Body goals diary

Body goals diary

Body goals diary

Body goals diary

Body goals diary

Body goals diary

About the author

C. T. Pam is not a physician, rather she is a regular person who has explored many avenues of eating healthy and finding a healthy lifestyle balance. After a car accident in 2010 left her unable to continue running, she found a work-life balance that has helped her maintain a healthy lifestyle. C. T. Pam has a B.A. in Political Science and Studio Art, an MBA with a entrepreneurship concentration and is currently pursuing a doctoral degree with a research focus in Entrepreneurship.

Book description

This book includes sound advice and facts regarding

- Introduction to weight management
- Choosing meal portions

While this book doesn't intend to tell the reader the best way to lead a healthy lifestyle, the author advises the reader to take away items that he or she can realistically achieve. You won't lose 50 pounds overnight, and you will have an opportunity to explore options that might benefit your physical, emotional and lifestyle needs. This book includes pages for the reader to record their goals and progress.

Volume 2 is an excerpt from Adopting a healthy lifestyle (1-884711-34-0)

Also available from Innovative Publishers

Introduction to the Paleo diet. (978-1884711466)

Introduction to the Paleo diet + 200 recipes (1884711820)

Love is… (978-1884711138)

Extreme Betrayal (978-1884711084)

Beware the Bumble Bee (978-1884711091)

Doing business with the U. S. government (978-1884711107)

Visit http://innovative-publishers.com for ordering information

Find us online @

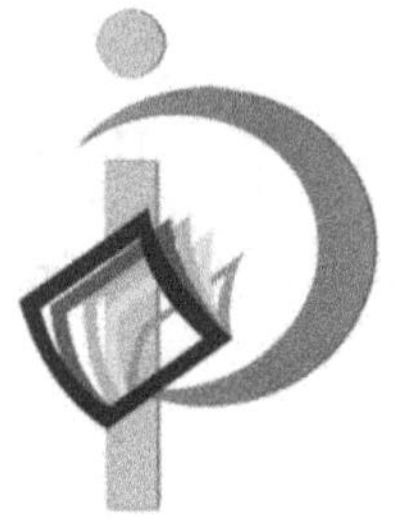

InnovaPub

www.innovative-publishers.com

pub@innovative-publishers.com

http://innovativepublishers.blogspot.com/

http://www.facebook.com/InnovativePublishers

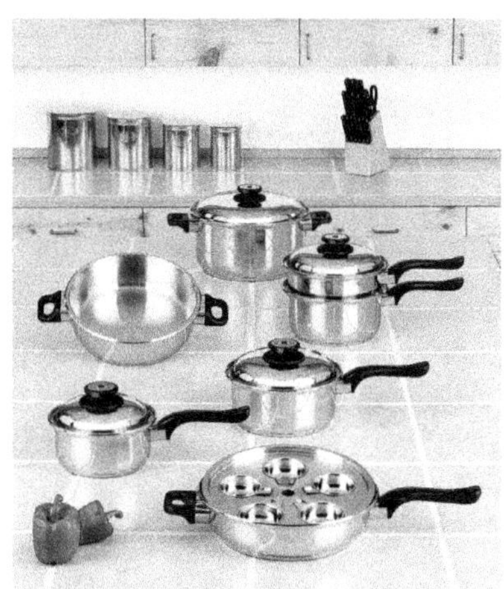

World's Finest™ 7-Ply Steam Control™ 17pc T304 Stainless Steel Cookware Set

Each piece is constructed of extra-heavy stainless steel and guaranteed to last a lifetime. Steam control valves make "waterless" cooking easy and the 7-ply construction spreads heat quickly and evenly, allowing one stack to cook. Cookware is also equipped with superbly styled phenolic handles resistant to heat, cold and detergents. Comes with a limited lifetime warranty. White box.

Suggested Retail Price : $2195.00

Item Number : GGKT17ULTRA

Set Contents

- 1.7Qt Covered Saucepan
- 2.5Qt Covered Saucepan
- 3.2Qt Covered Saucepan
- 7.5Qt Covered Roaster
- 11-3/8" Skillet, Double Boiler Unit With Capsule Bottom That You Can Also Use As An Extra 3Qt Saucepan
- 5 Egg Cups
- 5 Hole Utility Rack And High Dome Cover With Capsule Bottom So You Can Use As A Frypan
- Cover Fits Skillet Or Roaster

Features

- Extra-Heavy Stainless Steel Construction
- Heat-Resistant Phenolic Handles
- 7-Ply Construction

Limited Lifetime Warranty

» Estimated Case Weight : 36.55 Lbs.

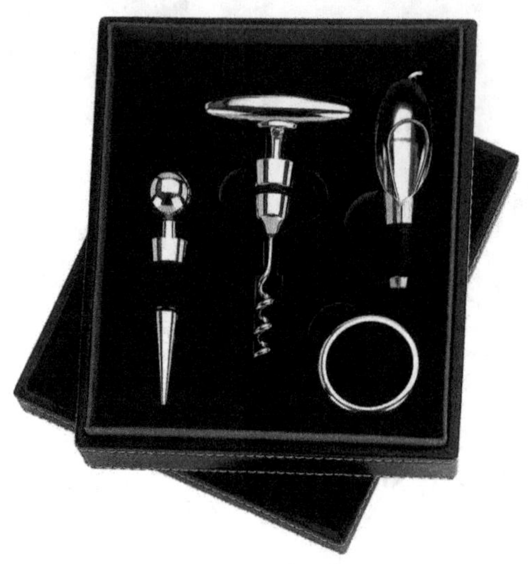

Wyndham House™ 4pc Wine Set in Storage Case

Wyndham House™ wine sets are a great compliment to any home bar, and are sure to add to the ease and elegance of wine presentations. Includes stainless steel wine spout, stainless steel wine ring, zinc alloy screw opener, and zinc alloy wine stopper. All enclosed in a 6-3/8" x 5-5/8" x 2-1/4" faux leather case.

Suggested Retail Price : $32.95

Next Ship Date : 01/05/2013

Item Number : GGKTWINE4

Features

- Stainless Steel Wine Spout
- Stainless Steel Wine Ring
- Zinc Alloy Screw Opener
- Zinc Alloy Wine Stopper
- 6-3/8" X 5-5/8" X 2-1/4" Faux Leather Case

Shipping Details

» Estimated Piece Weight : 1.10 Lbs.

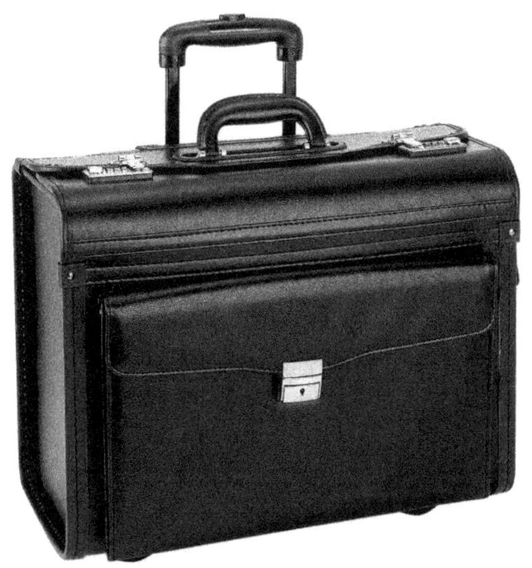

Embassy™ Sample/Pilot Case with Aluminum Trolley

Features PVC matte black exterior, rolling wheels, gunmetal combination locks, carrying handle, 2 exterior pockets, interior dividers, interior pockets, and pen holders. Measures 19" x 14" x 9".

Suggested Retail Price : $233.95

Number : BCPILOT3

Features

- Pvc Matte Black Exterior
- Rolling Wheels
- Gunmetal Combination Locks
- Carrying Handle
- 2 Exterior Side Pockets
- Interior Dividers & Pockets
- Pen Holders
- Measures 18" X 13" X 8"

Shipping Details

» Estimated Piece Weight : 8.70 Lbs.

To order products, go to the Innovative Publishers website and click Client specials. Clients receive up to 70% off the suggested retail price.

www.ingramcontent.com/pod-product-compliance
Lightning Source LLC
LaVergne TN
LVHW010107110826
845155LV00028B/526

* 9 7 8 1 8 8 4 7 1 1 7 0 1 *